Accelerated Learning:

How to Improve Your Memory

After 40, Never Forget a

Name or Date Again, and Stay

Young

I0134872

By John Gamberini

befitting its nature, it is presented without assurance regarding its prolonged validity or interim quality. Trademarks that are mentioned are done without written consent and can in no way be considered an endorsement from the trademark holder.

Medical Disclaimer

This book is not intended as a substitute for the medical advice of physicians. The reader should regularly consult a physician in matters relating to his/her health and particularly with respect to any symptoms that may require diagnosis or medical attention. Any recommendations given in this book are not a substitute for medical advice.

Table of Contents

Introduction

Welcome, and thanks for being here.

The following chapters will discuss how as you get older you can always continue to improve every facet of your life. When a person reaches the age of 40, they may think their best days are behind them and simply accept the upcoming mental decline. Aging is not the problem. Accepting defeat is. You do not have to accept anything just because your age is 40 or beyond.

There is no fountain of youth. This is common sense that many deny due to the fear of growing older and not being as sharp as they once were. Victories of yesterday lose value and expectations of upcoming victories seem less exciting. This is the cold and hard truth for many men after they surpass the age of 40.

It doesn't have to be that way though. Being tossed about by the winds of change is going to happen but there is no reason for a man to bow down and except being less then he once was as an inevitability. The mental aging process can be halted, and to an extent, reversed. You can fight back!

Just by downloading this book you have taken a powerful first step to reversing the mental aging process. Inside you will find a plethora of techniques and strategies that have been proven to keep the mind young, and for every technique, there will be exercises given to make sure that you receive the maximum benefit from applying them. As a quick note before we begin, these techniques do not require any prior training. You don't even have to have a "good memory" to benefit from them. There are no expensive tools or weird supplements needed either.

There are plenty of books on this subject on the market, thanks again for choosing this one! Every effort was made to ensure it is full of as much useful information as possible, please enjoy!

John Gamberini

Chapter 1: How Your Body Changes When You Turn 40

There is no one major culprit to blame when trying to place a bullseye upon the concept of memory loss and cognitive decay. A combination of factors all leads up to the decline of memory. Simply saying that "You are just getting older" is only a half-truth. Yes, these things happen as we age, but why? What is going on inside the body and brain that makes us slow down mentally as we move past the milestone of being 40?

Remember back to the last time you went through a great physiological change? It was probably all the way back in high school, and everyone told you that all the changes you were experiencing were hormones. Those hormones change again when you reach 40. Welcome back to school.

When talking about hormonal changes after 40 women and menopause typically get the unwanted spotlight. Andropause, the male equivalent, doesn't get talked about much but should be. This is also known as androgyne decline or testosterone deficiency. When younger, the average man will have testosterone levels at about over 1000 nanograms per deciliter. Then when he reaches 40, these levels drop around 1 percent per year. The lowering of testosterone levels will invariably have effects on how the brain functions. Fatigue, reduction of confidence, trouble sleeping, and the two bigger ones- memory loss and not being able to concentrate- are all reactions from testosterone levels lowering in the body.

As we grow older our neurons, unfortunately, decrease along with testosterone levels dropping lower. Testosterone can protect brain cells from damage, and also reduces the levels of a protein called beta-amyloid. Beta-amyloid, when unbalanced and unchecked, can wreak havoc on memory. The hippocampus, the area of our brains that has the most to do with retrieving and forming memories, breaks down. Blood flow to the brain will slow as age increases, which will have a maleficent effect on trying to produce new memories, as well as recalling old ones. Also, the grey matter (brain tissue made mostly of nerve cells and branching dendrites) will deteriorate and lead to a greater loss of memory functions. To be blunt, as we age our brains shrink and hormones become unbalanced.

However, it is also a scientific fact that at any age the brain can still make new cells. You can strengthen your brain, balance your hormones, and increase cognitive function across the board.

Testosterone replacement therapy (TRT) has become a medical strategy to counteract the natural process of testosterone decline. Human growth hormone (HGH) is another common phrase thrown around. What must be understood about hormones is that they are all supposed to benefit each other, find a balance, and join in unison. You are not supposed to pump yourself up with all sorts of hormones or shoot your testosterone levels through the roof. Doing so will only lead to an even greater imbalance, and thus, more memory and cognitive problems.

Testosterone and HGH are not the same hormones, and one must compliment the other. Keep that in mind if ever speaking to a doctor about these treatments. Testosterone is manufactured from the gonads, with smaller quantities coming from the adrenal glands. Yet HGH is manufactured from the pituitary gland inside the brain. Think of this as the lower body meting the higher and creating a cyclic balance. To find the proper balance and maintain it, is to keep your body and mind younger.

Although both TRT and HGH have their uses and share of benefactors, there is an equal amount of warnings relating to both of them. The jury is still out on the risks versus the rewards. The medical community is rapid with debate on both sides, and many tests regarding TRT and HGH are currently inconclusive. If speaking to a doctor about either of these, make sure you clearly understand exactly why they would recommend these treatments for you. Depending on your situation, HGH or TRT can cause more harm than good. Neither HGH or TRT should be mandatory for increasing cognitive functions.

Simply by reading these opening pages, you have begun the process of bettering your brain. Using scientific terminology here is not just used for accuracy, it has been a shadowed step to creating new cells in your brain and reversing the aging process.
Throughout the rest of this book, there will be several tips and exercises to keep this process going and deny the unwanted cognitive effects that come naturally with age.

Indeed, welcome back to school.

Chapter 2: Signs You May Be Experiencing Memory Loss

Everyone of any age can benefit from training their memory. For those who have reached the age of 40, it's safer to assume that your memory is in a state of decline then it is to just hope that it retains a razor-sharp edge. Many factors are going to be against your memory after your 40th birthday. There are several signs to keep an eye out for.

- Forgetting why you entered a room or started doing a task.
- Trouble recalling names.
- Mixing up numbers. These can be phone numbers, dates, or general information regarding your workplace.
- A growing fear of Alzheimer's or dementia.

- Blanking out on material that you know you have studied and learned.
- Trouble maintaining concentration.
- Misplacing items like car keys, your wallet, even not being able to find out where you parked your car.
- Needing to triple check everything to be sure that you did not forget something, and still missing a few details.
- Committing to a course, like learning a new language or memory training, and not seeing it through.
- A steady decrease in performance at work. Not just forgetting numbers, names, and appointments, but not being able to complete things you have done hundreds of times before as effectively as you once did.

If any of these happen to you infrequently then there is nothing to worry about. Slight slipups are common for even the most celebrated human minds. If these are common reoccurrences, however, then you are most likely already in a state of memory decline. The very first thing to do is NOT panic. That will only cause more stress and stifle your memory more. Recognize that there is a weakness in your memory, then you can begin the process of correcting it until it is better than ever before, even when you were younger and never had these problems.

Even if you don't suffer any of the listed issues regularly, the sooner you start training your memory the better.

A large number of things unseen and unrealized can be contributing to memory deficiency, and they can be happening to you right now. Again, do NOT panic. Remain calm as you take in this information. That is the best state of mind to be in for your memory to work to its fullest potential.

Four specific issues that often get overlooked when contemplating human memory and growing older are blood sugar, weight management, hearing, and even flossing.

Blood Sugar

If the blood sugar levels are above what they are supposed to be then they can cause damage to blood vessels in the brain. When blood flow to the brain becomes damaged, blocked, or reduced, not only will the entire brain (and then body) take a drastic blow to its health, but the memory will be substantially weakened.

A team of German researchers ran a study that analyzed over 100 people over a ten-year period. None of the participants had diabetes or any other impaired intolerance to glucose. They didn't have any prior issues with their memories or other cognitive impairments. The test was simple in practice. The participants had blood glucose tests done on them, then were required to perform various memory related tests, including recalling certain words less than an hour after hearing them. They also had their brains scanned, specifically the hippocampus, to see if there was any link between blood sugar levels and the part of the brain that is most responsible for forming and recalling memories.

The results they found were straight to the point. Those who had lower levels of blood sugar achieved higher scores on the memory tests then the others. They also discovered that the volume of the hippocampus decreased in relation to how high a person's blood sugar was. They also saw though diffusion tensor imaging that the structural integrity of the entire brain was lowered in people that had higher blood sugar levels. Their final conclusion to the test was, clinically speaking, even average blood sugar levels should be lowered. The lower your blood sugar, the better off it would be for your brain and memory.

It is wise to be aware of what your current blood sugar levels are. There are kits available to measure your blood sugar levels, or you may ask your doctor. Make sure you find out what your current level is.

Weight Management

The body mass index (BMI) is used to determine if someone is underweight or over. Using BMI is not a direct measure of body fat. It is a weight-to-height ratio that lets someone know if they are the proper weight for their height. If you were to go see a doctor regarding your memory one of the first things they will look into is your BMI. If someone's BMI is less than 18.5 then they are underweight. If the BMI is over 25, they are overweight.

According to the University of Arizona, having a higher BMI (and remember that 25 is the max number to not exceed) can cause a negative effect to overall brain health. All the reasoning behind this is unknown, but the culprit can most likely be traced back to inflammation. Even if only the brain is inflamed alone it can cause a negative impact on all cognitive functioning. It does not take a strong imagination to see why this would be the case. Just think back to any time you have had an infection, or just a swelling, in some part of your body. Now alter those same sensations to the brain and seeing how an inflamed brain can affect cognitive ability should be easy to understand. This directly relates to BMI. The higher count that your BMI is, the more likely that there will be inflammation somewhere in your body.

Inflammation can be measured via C-reactive protein (CRP). The study done at the university of Arizona found a direct link between CRP, BMI, and declining brain functioning. The higher someone's BMI was, the more their CRP levels changed. The higher their CRP (used to measure inflammation) became, the more they saw a decrease in a participant's memory and executive brain functioning.

Out of all the debates that exist within any conversation regarding health, weight management is always at the top of the list. It just so happens that keeping BMI under 25 is not just good for your physical body, but also your mind as well. Find out what your BMI currently is.

Hearing

Neuroplasticity is the brain's ability to create new synaptic connections or reorganize them. This process takes place every time new knowledge is gained and learned. How well you can hear has a direct correlation to this process of neuroplasticity.

Hearing only diminishes over time. This will happen naturally with age. As hearing gets worse the brain will induce a process of neuroplasticity called cross-modal cortical reorganization. This happens once an area of the brain that is dedicated to one of our five senses (in this case hearing) starts to diminish. When that happens, the brain will have to compensate for the weakened area and have one of the other sensory faculties start to carry the extra weight. Think of it like this; when your hearing starts to go, places in your brain that are used to handling vision, touch, olfactory, or taste will begin to also take on the extra tasks of your hearing. This sort of rewiring of the brain can cause many disruptions of sensation and confuse the brain's ability to work at its fullest potential. The worse your hearing is, the easier it is for your brain to mix a signal and become confused.

Even more, when the brain cannot correctly process sound, it also can't interpret speech as it should. This will lead to another case of neuroplasticity gone wrong. The brain will rewire itself to better understand sound and speech, but by doing so its higher centers that we use to make tough and fast decisions will be distracted by carrying the extra cargo of deciphering sound and interpreting speech. These higher centers of the brain should be helping us to recall things faster and remember everything we need to so that we can navigate our world correctly. Instead, they are focused on hearing and not doing their true jobs or serving their original purpose.

The earlier hearing loss is detected the sooner you can get to work preventing further decay. Get a hearing test as soon as you can.

Dental Hygiene

There is a direct link between oral health and dementia. *Porphyromonas gingivalis* is a bacterium that can exit the mouth and make its way into the brain. This can happen from brushing your teeth or even just by chewing food. Even minor dental work can cause this bacterium to slip in where it should never be. All the hard data on this link is still being discovered, but one thing can be certain, gums can become inflamed. As we have already covered, any inflammation can start a snowball effect through the rest of the body and over time can affect the brain.

Although simple daily things like eating and brushing can lead to *Porphyromonas gingivalis* going where it shouldn't, flossing has not been shown to have the same negative effects. We are not condoning skipping the dentist appointments or brushing your teeth and are certainly not telling you to starve yourself. Daily flossing, twice a day, should be added to your daily oral regimen if it is not already. Whatever bacteria gets loosened around in the mouth from built up plaque can be removed safely from flossing. Also, be sure to keep up your regular visits to the dentist. As each year passes by more and more information is being unveiled relating between oral and brain health. Try to keep up on any plaque buildup that may be happening.

Mental Health

Knowing your blood sugar levels, BMI, having your hearing checked, and flossing daily are only four of the different aspects that can affect your cognition and memory. There are other items you should be aware of.

Depression

Being depressed is never a state of mind anyone would ever want to enter. Aside from the obvious information about depression, it has also been proven to have a direct effect on short-term memory loss. Knowing that, if someone who is depressed finds a way to exit that frame of mind then their memory should improve. Depression does not, on its own, have an effect on long-term or procedural memory. When depressed, your brain will simply not want to retain the memories it forms during such a dour state.

New memories will not imprint as well and become forgotten. This is the minds self-defense mechanism to avoid becoming more depressed. Also, when depressed the brain will be stuck in a state of confusion perpetually.

With depression will follow different levels of anxiety and stress. Any combination of these three things will impair making proper decisions and fill the mind with opaque clouds of fogginess.

Two separate studies were done, one in 2013 and another in 2015. Both of these tests were the same concept where a group of people who were suffering from depression were asked to identify objects on a screen. These objects were items that were either identical or similar to objects that they had been shown before. Both studies showed the same exact results; people suffering from depression could not identify most of the objects they were shown. This was just more proof that depression has a negative effect on short-term memory.

How to Build the Proper Frame of Mind for Optimal Memory Health

While reading this chapter you have been told NOT to panic. That is valuable advice that you should take away and use at all times, not just in regard to memory but in every situation and circumstance that you will ever face always try your best to NOT panic. Not panicking is a necessity to remembering the smallest details of whatever you may be going through.

Before any living creature has ever done any action or moved a muscle, there was a thought in the mind that existed if even for a split-second before the action happened in the world outside their mind. When in a state of panic, the mind is not thinking clearly enough to perform the proper action after having a thought, whatever that action may be. This is not a message of the metaphysical or experimental psychology. This is very practical advice that can all be boiled down to one specific point- you have to build the right mindset.

When first facing a problem, everything seems like a losing battle. Challenges, especially regarding health, can give of the essence of feeling like you are all alone even if you're not. Most likely you're not alone, but even if you are or just feel that way, you can reverse the mental aging process and defeat the cowardly crimson jackal of memory loss. It has been said that the only thing any man ever needs to be better than is their former selves. If you truly believe that you cannot win, that you are never going to strengthen your memory, then you are correct. You have already waved the white flag of submission. Yet, if you change that mindset into one that is conducive to victory, learn what the problem is, take the proper steps, then you can keep the mind young.

See yourself as a winner in everyday life! Whatever it is that you do at your job, in your spare time, with friends or family, sports, video games, painting a room, watching television, envision yourself doing it better then you ever have before.

Before doing any tasks or stepping out of the house, envision yourself accomplishing what you are setting out to do. If you are going to go to the dentist, imagine yourself coming back home with a bright smile. If you are going to watch television, envision yourself having a great time watching it. If you want to increase your memory, envision yourself recalling information when you need it. There is never a task where you should envision yourself failing, nor is there any action so small it should not be visualized and surrounded with success beforehand.

When facing challenges, or anything else, never focus on the negative. What you focus on is where your attention is going to go. While someone is focusing on the negative there can be positivity that is passing them by and they would not even notice.

The Navy Seal Trick

It does not matter what tiny achievements you accomplish during your day. When trying to tear down your old foundations and replace them with new ones, you have to remove as much negativity from your mental sphere as you can.

This is not just simple positive affirmations. Positive affirmations do have their place, and they are good practices to start instilling in your life, but there is also a logic to these concepts that often gets skirted past far too quickly. The point off repeating a positive affirmation is to instill the belief of what you are repeating into the core of your being. It's to rewrite your own brain chemistry, to be the self-appointed neuro surgeon and steer the process of neuroplasticity exactly where you want it to go.

When learning something new and neuroplasticity takes places your brain introduces a variety of chemicals, and these chemicals collect together to send out signals through the rest of the brain and body. This is how new information is gained and stored in our brains. When this happens, the brain rewires itself, and certain pieces of it will even change in shape. Just by learning something new, you are literally altering the shape and mechanism of your brain. This is partly how habits can develop. When your brain is a certain shape and used to sending out a series of specific signals, it will continue to do what it has always done before. We are creatures of habit and that includes our brains. If you are stuck in a negative loop and only focusing on your losses, troubles, problems, and challenges, then you have taught your brain to have a defeatist attitude, and being a product of habit, that defeatist nature will continue to play over and over again.

All the specifics of exactly how human memory works is still up in the air and will continue to be for some time to come. Many brilliant people have tried to understand the great mystery of the human mind, consciousness, and memory for eons and we have only scratched the tip of the iceberg. We know memories form in the hippocampus, but where they are stored is an unanswered question. Currently, most of the signs are pointing to the idea that memories are not stored simply in one location but are allocated into different parts of the brain for wherever they fit best. This would make sense. If a certain smell triggered a specific memory, but a certain sound triggered another, then it can be assumed that one memory would be somewhere closer to your olfactory receptors while another would be closer to the areas that are responsible for hearing and interpreting sound.

There isn't one magic trick to alter the way you think from a negative and defeatist outlook to one that is more positive. Yet, remembering your successes is as close as you are going to get to finding a one size fits all trick to rewire your brain into how you want it to operate.

As your age increases and your memory starts to wane, it is going to be extra important on what you CHOOSE to remember. What you think about you bring about and selecting the right types of memories to hold onto and figuring out which are the correct ones to discard, will be very valuable to transforming the vicious cycle of how you think into one that brings the results you want to happen.

If you are only thinking of your troubles and losses then you are wiring your brain to assume, accept, and be more conducive to recreating negative circumstances. If you focus on your victories, if you continuously tell your brain to rewire itself into something that is more conducive to positivity and productivity, then your brain will do that instead.

The best way to get started switching your brain from something that focuses on the negative and forgets more then it remembers is to write down and remember your successes.

Take a few minutes out of your day to recall your greatest achievements, whatever they may be. It doesn't matter if they happened years ago or yesterday. Focus on those accomplishments that gave you the most fulfillment. Focusing on those will not only rewire your brain to repeat such accomplishments but will increase your concentration.

Live in the now of your current successes. By downloading this book and reading this far you have taken a big step towards bettering yourself, and that's a positive trait that you should focus on. If there were any words or scientific concepts that you may not have understood, look them up and take a little bit of time to do more research (I recommend typing *H.M and the hippocampus* in a search engine). Then be proud of doing such a thing and recognize it as another success.

Did you leave the house today and make it to an appointment on time? Did you find a good parking space? Have you learned anything new? Did you hold open a door for someone, pay bills, cook breakfast? Anything remotely positive is what you should be focusing on instead of worrying what may or may not come. There is no gain that cannot be grown into another gain, no victory that is not worth celebrating, no success that should go unrecognized. It really doesn't matter how small these victories seem. As you continue to do this you may see those tiny success stories snowball into powerful boulders and crush the former defeatist notion that may weaken your mental faculties, including memory, to being with.

Then start writing them down. If you already have a journal and make daily entrees then you have a leg up on the battle. If you do not, get one. Don't just remember your success, jot them down to review later when you may be feeling down or forgetful.

When you write something down you are less likely to forget about it later. Writing things down is more engaging for the entire body, and mind, then simply absorbing information. This is why taking notes is considered one of the best forms of studying. It's not just to look things up later but also to solidify what you are doing. You may even want to kick this concept up to the next level and reread some of this book and bust out the pen and paper, then start taking notes. After doing so, read this book again up to this current chapter. You will probably notice that you already can recall most of the information faster than before. This should happen not just because of repetition, but because you were taking the extra step to engage both your body and mind in the same activity at the same time.

Even the toughest and most mentally fit people on the planet use these techniques. The Navy Seals are known to both journal and write down their victories, not just the ones they win out on the field. The concept that the Navy Seals need to rely upon is keeping their spirits high (staying more positive) even during the most daunting of circumstances. No Navy Seal would claim that before going into training or a mission that they had instilled themselves with a defeatist attitude. That would only bring ruin, failure, possibly death. The Navy Seals are often placed in situations where they MUST win no matter the cost.

How can this strong mindset be kept, how to remember and focus on the successes when there may just not be that much going on to feel proud or thankful over? The solution would be to think smaller instead of bigger. That's why it has been emphasized to remember and write down your successes no matter what they may be. They don't even need to be victories brought on by your own actions.

It is common for a Navy Seal to write down three things that they found success with inside their journals every day. Imagine the most boring and uneventful day you can. It may seem like there just is not any victory to find, but then when it comes time to jot things down in your journal, it winds up looking something like this...

- *After the rain stopped there was a cool breeze blowing through the air.*
- *When I sat down to drink my tea, it tasted just right and cleared my head.*
- *I took the time to write down in my journal.*

Those quaint little entries will make a stronger impact then you think. Make it a daily practice to write down your success. Doing so will bring confidence and improve your ability to retain facts, like a Navy Seal.

The key word to the phrase "Remembering your successes" is *remembering.* If you take the time to tell your brain that success is what you want to remember and remain aware that the brain will rewire itself through neuroplasticity, you are not only increasing your concentration, reshaping your state of mind into one more conducive to success, but also telling your brain to start increasing your capacity for remembering overall! By doing this you will be uploading new software into the computer known as your brain and readjusting all its properties to be less forgetful. The human brain is the world's most powerful machine and all you have to learn is how to operate it correctly.

Getting Proper Nutrition without Breaking the Bank

What you put inside of your body will have a great effect on how well you function. Below is a list of foods that will help to boost memory and concentration.

- **Nuts:** One ounce of nuts a day will give you all the amino acids that you need to increase your focus. They are also chalked full of vitamin E which has been proven to halt the decreasing of cognitive functions.
- **Dark Chocolate:** Avoid the sugary chocolates. Dark chocolate can release dopamine and serotonin into the blood stream which will help to relax the mind. It also contains trace amounts of caffeine which can help to boost mental awareness. A small handful or even one square piece should be all you need.

- **Flax Seed:** Flax seed has B-vitamins and Omega-3 fatty acids which can help to boost both focus and mental clarity.
- **Blueberries:** The antioxidants in blueberries can increase both blood flow and oxygen to the brain. They have also been proven to boost focus.
- **Avocados:** Avocados have also been proven to increase proper blood flow to the brain.
- **Green Tea:** Another great way to get a little bit of caffeine to help increase mental awareness is through Green tea. It has also been proven to increase focus.
- **Water:** Every part of your body, including the brain, depends on water. Every aspect of brain function will be improved by drinking water.
- **Fish:** Herring, sardines, mackerel, salmon, trout, and kipper contain Omega-3 fatty acids which will boost your memory. If there is a miracle food for memory, it's fish.

- **Vegetables:** Leafy greened veggies have folic acids, B-vitamins and antioxidants, all of which will increase your memory and overall brain performance. Add lots of leafy green vegetables to your diet.

The #1 Supplement for Memory Loss

Having a vitamin B-12 deficiency has been proven to lead to memory loss. To avoid this, make sure that you are getting enough of the vitamin on a regular basis. This is one of the most common factors that lead to memory problems and it is also very easily solved. Just take a vitamin B-12 supplement and you should be on your way overriding this problem. B-12 is the most important supplement for optimal memory performance at any age.

It is important to keep in mind that the world of vitamins and supplements has become a cutthroat industry. There is a plethora of competition and trickery involved. You should not just be buying the cheapest, or the most expensive. Do a little bit of research before buying vitamin B-12 and find out which one works best for you.

Chapter 3: Cultivating a Daily Routine and Habits

The actions we do while awake and the way we sleep at night are intimately connected to how our brains work for us as individuals. Getting into a proper rhythm with your daily habits and sleep will help to balance both the body and mind and improve your mental capacity in every area of life.

Daily Habits

There are a number of things you can introduce into your daily life that will have a positive effect on how your brain functions.

- **Rubik's Cube:** Trying to solve a Rubik's cube can help increase concentration. It also instills patience and quiets down the mind from whatever chatter going on in the background.

Getting into the habit of becoming a problem solver will only help to increase all of your mental conditioning.

- **Chopsticks:** When using chopsticks, you are forcing your brain to be more aware of what you are doing and increasing your concentration. You will also be installing subconscious automated memories into yourself, increasing your mental capacity without realizing it. You'll be learning a new etiquette when eating and trying to remember the rules of the etiquette will be another exercise in boosting your memory.

- **Meditation:** Meditation is used to increase memory, focus, clear the mind, and increase awareness. No one has ever said that meditation has made their life worse or caused them to be more forgetful and concentrate less. If you are new to the practice start by doing it for five minutes every day. Focus on either your breath or picture an image in your head and try to hold it. If you can't find the time to meditate then at least find a calm space to visit once a day and just go there to relax.

- **Set Small Goals Every Day:** Even something as simple as getting out of bed by 7:30 or reading a single chapter of a book. Make a list the night before of small goals to reach.

How to Build a Consistent Sleep Routine

While we sleep the body repairs itself from the cells of our flesh all the way to the nerves of our brains. Nothing is more recuperative for the body and mind then sleep. Sleep is often something many people take for granted until they start to have problems with it. Think of sleep as natures repair shop, when as you slumber, both your body and mind can receive the proper maintenance.

If you are not getting the right amount of sleep, your memory is destined to deteriorate. Be aware that the more energy you use during the day or the more stress you have to endure will mean that you may need some extra time sleeping.

If you are having problems getting your sleep cycle to how you want it to be then you may need to reset your sleep. Humans have a built-in internal clock known as the circadian clock. Since we have fluctuating schedules, we lose track of our circadian clock. But it's possible to get it back on track.

- **Stick to a schedule:** Go to sleep at the same time every night. Keep a schedule in your daily activities as well. Eat at the same times, expend energy at the same times, and anything else you can think of.
- **Watch your caffeine intake:** Do not consume any caffeine six hours before bedtime.
- **Exercise:** This will expend energy so when you hit the hay your body is ready to sleep. It will also help your body to repair more during the night.
- **No electrical lights:** Turn down the screens and any blue lights that may be in the room.
- **Get a routine before bed:** Brushing your teeth, meditating, stretching, journaling, anything that's calming you should do every night before

bed. Setting up a routine will let your body know that it is time to wind down sleep.

The Hidden Dangers of Doctor Prescribed Sleeping Pills

Many who have problems sleeping find reliance upon over-the-counter medication. Not only can sleeping pills become addictive but they have been shown to have a negative effect on brain health, specifically memory. What you really want to watch out for is any sleep aid that contains the ingredient diphenhydramine. Diphenhydramine can make you foggy headed after waking up. It can also lead to difficulty concentrating and has even been directly linked to short-term memory loss. Try to use the previous methods mentioned instead of using sleeping pills.

Chapter 4: Memory Training for Over 40s

You are just about ready to get into the practical training methods used to strengthen your memory. Before that, though it should be clarified why there are so many different memory techniques. Truth be told, they are all similar and only separated from their origins. Since the dawn of time man has been trying to unravel the mystery behind memory and become better at utilizing it. Because of this, various people from different epochs and cultures have devised their own particular methods. Yet, the rules behind memory are always the same. Memory is associative; everything that is introduced to the brain is compared to something else like it or completely opposite of it. Due to every technique following the same paradigm of association, similarities will be apparent, yet they are all worth practicing. The more tools you have, the more work you can get done.

STM and LTM

You have seen the terms "short-term" (STM) and "long-term" (LTM) memory throughout this book. There are some key differences regarding these two forms of memory worth noting.

STM has 3 major aspects connected to it.

- **Encoding:** Encoding takes place within LTM and well as STM. Think of a ball of clay that you can press your finger into. If you press lightly and only for a second, then the clay may not hold onto to the image of your finger for long and reset back to normal. But if you press down harder and longer, then the image of your finger will remain longer, possibly permanently. This is similar to how encoding works. You may also refer to encoding as imprinting. The type of encoding will differ depending on sensory input.

- **Short Duration:** Whatever information enters the brain and only encodes in STM will be lost rather quickly. The duration of time needed to pass before it disappears may vary, but even a slight distraction can cause you to forget all about it. Certain studies have shown that the time length before forgetting in STM may only be between 15-30 seconds long.

- **Small Capacity:** The STM of an average adult can only hold between 5-9 items at a time. For most people, they can hold 7 items. Think of STM as only having so many slots that can be filled up. Then those slots are emptied out, so other memories can find storage within them.

The first thing that happens when forming a memory is encoding. The second stage of memory is STM, and the final stage is LTM.

Before encoding even begins someone will have to give their attention to something. After giving attention to what the person finds interest in, the item will be formed into a mental construct, so it can be encoded inside the brain. Then later it can be recalled from either STM or LTM. The strength of the sensory (whether something was loud, bright, noticeable) will help determine how deeply the item is encoded. One of the key factors in making a sensory impulse stronger is whether or not emotion is attached to the forming memory. Most likely the most memorable moments in your life had emotions, positive and negative, attached to them.

After a memory is encoded in the brain, it will make its way to the hippocampus. Once it arrives there it is up to the hippocampus to determine if the memory should remain slotted in STM or placed deeper in LTM. The hippocampus will compare the new memory to older ones when figuring out where to allocate the new memory, to check how important it is and whether it is worth holding onto. If it does determine to allocate the new memory to LTM then...the rest is unknown. As stated earlier it is most likely that memories allocated to LTM are placed within different areas of the brain, but more information is needed before that can be declared as fact. As science advances more will be made clear on the mystery of the human mind and memory allocation, but that day may not come for a long time.

There are 4 different types of encoding that happen when a new memory is forming.

- **Acoustic:** Processing and recording of sounds.
- **Visual:** Recording of all visual stimulus.
- **Tactile:** Recording how something feels to touch.
- **Semantic:** Recording sensory input related to context. This is LTM only.

Besides the different ways the brain encodes and the different types of STM, LTM also has some distinct aspects.

- **Semantic:** Also listed above. This is a declarative and factual memory about your environment and the world. An example would be; the capital of Australia is Canberra.
- **Procedural:** This is non-declarative, as in motor skills and knowing how to do something. An example would be playing the piano.
- **Episodic:** This is declarative and also connects to conscious thinking. It has to do with remembering a sequence of events, like meeting someone new or moving to a new home.

Recall

First memories are encoded, then stored, and then later they can be recalled. There are three different types of ways memories are recalled

- **Free Recall:** This is when a memory is recalled without any extra help. If someone asks you something, the answer comes to you without needing a technique. This is most likely to happen for memories that are strongly imprinted or happened recently.

- **Cued Recall:** This is when something reminds you of something else. Like seeing an image and then recalling what the image reminds you of.

- **Serial Recall:** This is recalling information in the correct order that it was originally presented. This is used every time you speak, repeat something that was heard, or even when using a recipe or performing a dance sequence.

The 60 Year Old TV Trick

This is the final thing you should understand before diving into the training. There is nothing more valuable to your memory and state of mind then the power of "thinking in images". We are not born with a determined language. If someone is deaf or mute, they lack the linguistic abilities that others have. Before the first man walked upon the earth, there was no human speech. Images were the original language and are still a powerful tool for teaching your mind what is and is not important. Whatever self-limiting things you think of yourself (like saying "I'm going to forget that") can be overridden by replacing it with an image of the outcome you want.

Have you ever heard of the name Harry Lorayne? He was a mentalist and considered a master of memory that was first introduced to the world at large on the television show *"I've got a secret"* back in 1958. As the audience members (500 of them) were filling into the building, Mr. Lorayne asked every one of them their names. Later, after the show had been going on for several minutes, he was asked to randomly recall the audience members names. He didn't forget any of them, even when the host of the show decided to challenge him further by tossing a ball into the audience and having random people catch it. Harry Lorayne was asked to say the name of all the different people who caught the ball, and even then he still named everyone correctly.

To quote Mr. Lorayne... "The cliché I've heard all my life is, I recognize your face, but I can't remember your name. You know, in my long and happily successful career I've never heard it said the other way around."

What was the major secret to Harry Lorayne's amazing memory? Associating names, numbers, and everything else with images. Seeing as imagery is the original and silent language that preexists all humanity, this makes perfect sense. Imagery exists before language and speech, so it is only a natural course for our brains to cling to an image first and then associate a word with it. When meeting someone new, first take a look at their face and find something particular about it. A really easy example would be someone with green eyes. If their name is Mr. Green, then remembering them will not be difficult. If the name is more complicated though, you will need to be more creative.

As you begin practicing the different mnemonic techniques these mystifying concepts will become clearer to you. Practice makes perfect.

Now it is time for the training. Be aware that you will have to practice these systems every day or you will not get the results that you want. Things may seem slow at first as if your memory is not improving at the rate that you want it to. This will only be an illusion though. The improvement of your memory will be gradual but if you stick with it and practice every day then you will start to forget things less without even realizing it at first. Most likely, you won't see the true power of these techniques until someone points out to you how good your memory is.

Now it is time to start training.

Pegging

The pegging, or hook, the system is all about associating certain words to numbers. Think of "pegging" as in the concept of linking one item to another. Stop for a moment and don't think as objects or numbers as what they are, but just think of them as general data or information. You are hanging one piece of information onto another. Take a hat and a hat rack as an example. One piece of information is the hat, and the other is the rack. You are only placing the information of the hat, onto the peg of the rack, so you can grab it later when you need to remember it. When you dive into the peg list, this will start to make more sense to you.

Memory pegs are used for memorizing a list of numbers in a sequential order, but you are supposed to attach (or hang) images of objects onto the numbers- so it is really just using numbers to remember a series of objects. The peg will be an image in your mind that you hang the number onto. This will come in very handy next time you go out shopping at the supermarket or any other store. When trying to remember a series of different items that you need to buy, just trying to recall every item on the list may seem quite daunting to remember. That's why the first thing you will have to do is create a "peg list". For each number on the list, you will want to create a mental image that helps you to recall one for the other.

This may seem a bit odd when first discovering it but don't worry, you only have to memorize your peg list one time, then you can apply it to a variety of different situations. One study showed that participants could memorize six separate lists of objects while only using the same peg list!

There are many different types of memory peg systems. The one that seems to work best for most people is the rhyming pegs. Rhyming is one of the easiest ways to recall two things at the same time because the similar sounds of the words are a natural association. Since when new memories enter the hippocampus, and the hippocampus will compare new memories to older ones, your hippocampus will most likely store the new rhyming memory into your LTM. When your hippocampus hears a rhyme, it will automatically assume the new memory is similar to an older one and hold onto it.

To get you started practicing this take a look at the example peg list. First, there will be a number, and then an object that you will associate with that number. When reading the list first say the number, and then envision the object following it. For example, after saying the number *one*, envision the *sun* in the sky and keep in mind that earth only has *one sun*. Every time you need to remember to buy only *one* of something (let's say a skillet) you will want to replace the *sun* with that object. So, when remembering to buy only *one* skillet, instead of seeing the *sun* up there in the blue sky, you will see a skillet hanging above the earth. This may seem absurd, but to quote Mr. Lorayne again...

"Making the pictures ridiculous is what enables you to really see them; a logical picture is usually to vague."

Here is your example peg list.

- One = Sun (our planet only has one sun)
- Two = Shoe (we wear two pairs of shoes)
- 3 = Tree (envision the tree with three branches)
- 4 = Score (Think of the score of a game being won by 4 points)
- 5 = Hive (think of five bees going into their hive)

- 6 = Sticks (imagine six sticks bunched together)
- 7 = Heaven (as in the phrase 7th heaven)
- 8 = Skate (as in figure 8's)
- 9 = Shine (Envision the number 9 glowing bright)
- 10 = Men (Imagine ten men working together)

You may use this peg list or create your own. If you do create your own then make sure that the words you chose to rhyme with the numbers. Either use this list or create your own before the next time you go out shopping, as this will be your first mnemonic exercise. Don't carry the peg list around with you though, memorize it first. If your memory is already wayward, then take extra time to make sure you memorize your peg list. The start may be difficult, but the results will pay off in dividends after you get going. As with many challenges, the beginning is the hardest part.

If it helps, get out a piece of paper and write the number down, then draw next to it a picture (it doesn't matter how crude it may look) of the object. So, write down the number 2, and then draw a pair of shoes next to the number 2. Like the Navy Seal technique of writing things down, drawing will also engage your body and mind together and help to remember why you drew the image in the first place. In fact, as you make journal entries of your day you may even want to start drawing in it as well since that is another way to empower your memory.

When creating your peg list or using this books example, make sure the images associated with the numbers are detailed. Going back to having the number 2 being pegged with shoes, make sure you see what color the shoes are. You may even want to make them separate colors, one white and the other black. Take extra effort to create the details of the laces in your mind. Are the laces long or short, what color are the laces? Use this attention to detail for every item on your peg list so you can recall them easier as time goes on.

When memorizing your peg list read each number and the object linked to it aloud. Since the words rhyme (*two* and *shoe)* saying them aloud will help to sink them deeper into your brain. Then focus on the object in your mind until you see it clearly. Just by doing this you will be practicing concentration. Do this several times with your own peg list or the example we have given you. Continue to go over it from top to bottom again and again before moving onto the next step. After you are confident that you can remember all the associations on your peg list, you are ready to do some practical field work and put your memory to the test.

Memory Enhancement Exercise 1: Shopping with a Peg List

The following description of the exercise is only an example. It involves shopping at the grocery store in the real world. Next time you go out shopping alter this example to fit your needs. Don't just go out and buy the items on this example list verbatim, buy what you really want and need in your life.

Say you are going to the store and need to buy the following items; a loaf of bread, milk, a dozen eggs, 2 carrots, butter, and 3 cans of soup. Before stepping out of your house you are going to place a number on each item and peg an image to link the number and item.

You need one loaf of bread. *One* rhymes with *sun.* First, imagine the *sun* in the sky, and then stick a loaf of bread directly in the middle of the sun.

You also need milk. Now it may get tricky so pay attention. You only need *one* gallon of milk, but it is number *two* on your list. Again, imagine the *sun* so you will remember that you only need to buy *one* of something (in this case milk). But, since *two* rhymes with *shoe*, instead of placing milk in the center of the sun, place *two shoes* that are overflowing with milk inside them in the center of the sun. Yes, the image is absurd but that will help you to not forget it.

Then you will need a dozen eggs. The number twelve was not on the example peg list, and that was done by design to show you a real-life example. When shopping in the real world you are probably going to come across situations that will not follow the list exactly. However, all you have to do is expand the concept a little further and you will be fine. *Shelve* rhymes with *twelve*, so when looking over your shopping list and seeing a dozen eggs listed, imagine *twelve shelves* filled with eggs. But, since it is also number *three* on your list, and *three* rhymes with *tree*, imagine *three trees*, all with *three* branches each surrounding the *twelve* *shelves* filled with eggs. Again, the more absurd the image the more likely you are to remember it.

Next is *two* carrots, but they are number *four* on your list. So, imagine *two shoes* with carrots sticking out of them and place them on a *score* board. *Score* rhymes with *four* as shown in the example list.

Number *five* on your list is butter. *Five* rhymes with *hive*, but you only need *one* package of butter. Imagine the *sun* again, but place in the center of it a *hive* with butter oozing out of it.

Last on your shopping list is *three* cans of soup. Since this is number *six* on your list, imagine *six* branches of *sticks* all pointing to *three trees* which have *three* soup cans growing from them.

This exercise may seem difficult but once you start doing it you should come to realize that you successfully acquired everything on your shopping list. Then go home and jot down in your journal that you successfully bought everything you needed. Always write down your successes.

Memory Enhancement Exercise 2: Random Questions

Ask someone you know to write down a list of random objects labeled 1-20. Have them read the list to you just once, then separate for a half hour. While they are reading the list to you make sure to use pegging and visualize everything they tell you. After a half hour have them come back and ask you three questions.

"What was number six...what was number nine...what was number fifteen?"

It is up to them, not you, to pick which numbers from the list to ask. All you are supposed to do is recite the object that was connected to the number. If you don't do so well, don't lose heart. Try again the next day, then the next, and so on until you can answer every question they ask correctly.

The World Champion Major Method

The Major Method also works on the premise that images are easier to recall then words or numbers. The Major Method primarily works for memorizing a string of numbers. The basic premise is that you are going to convert the numbers into hard constants sounds. An example may look like this, using the number zero.

0 = z/s/c (soft).

This is known as an arbitrary association, meaning it seems random. The word zero begins with a "Z". The letters "Z" and "S" both have *zero* vertical strokes (same as the numeral 0). To minimize the arbitrariness (randomness) of this concept, associate an image with the number *zero*. A popular image for understating this concept is a snake eating its own tail (also known as *Ouroboros*- if you want your mind blown do some research on the symbol). The image of a snake eating its own tail is in the shape of the number *zero* (0). Snakes also hiss, which is a sound that is associated with the letters "S" and "Z".

Another example would be using the number 1.

1 = T/D.

Both "T" and "D" only have *one* vertical stroke, same as the numeral 1. The previous sentence is very important- read it again. Now let's skip ahead a bit and cover the Major Method's use for the number 2.

2 = "N".

The letter "N" has *2* vertical strokes. But what about the numbers 3 and 4?

3 = "M".

4= "R".

"M" has 3 vertical strokes, and when turned sideways it looks like a 3. Are you starting to see how there is a natural and unnoticed association between certain letters and numbers yet? Not everything involves strokes though. In the case of 4 = "R", "R" is the final letter when spelling *four*, and if you place them side by side (4R) then you will notice that they are almost inverted images of each other.

Now let's go back to 1 = T/D.

You are going to want to create a letter-sound association and to do that you will need to connect and image to the thought of 1 = T/D. Use either a toad or a dog. Now, to make things less arbitrary and random you don't want to just link the number 1 and letters T/D to any toad or dog. Use something clear and specific, like a dog you had during childhood or a toad you saw in a movie. The point of this is to convert these arbitrary associations into non-arbitrary ones, to make them less random and personalize them to your unique brain.

Now, we know that 2 = "N" and 4= "R". Let's use that to take a look at the number 42 and associate it with a word.

When trying to remember the number 42, you can use the Major Method to convert the number into the word *rain.* Whenever you will need to remember the number 42, you will think of and visualize rain. When you need to remember the number 1, you will visualize a dog or toad.

Keep in mind that when using the Major Method, you will not be using any vowels and only placing them in as filler. The "a" and "i" in the word *rain* are the fillers.

Let's assume that you had to go and purchase one (1) 42-inch ladder. Before going out to purchase it, envision a dog (1= "D") running in the rain (2 = "N" and 4 = "R"). When you get to the store you will probably remember what you went there for.

Admittedly this seems very confusing at first but if you spend a few minutes practicing everyday it will all start to come naturally to you.

Memory Enhancement Exercise 3: Creating Your Own List

Due to the fact that the Major Method can be difficult, you will want to start out with an easy exercise at first. There are many different sources that you can look up to find the Major Method list. That will be something that you will have to look up, but not right away.

First, you are going to get a piece of paper and write down the numbers 1-9. For every number, you are going to write the name of an object next to it. These objects are all going to have to be specific things that you are familiar with. Don't just write "dog" next to the number 1. Write a specific sort of dog that you used to or still know. Do this for every number. After compiling it, study the list very carefully. Then put it away.

The following day you are to pull out the list and before looking at it, just try to remember the images you allotted for the numbers 1-5. Take your time until you recall each image, or until you are sure you won't remember them. Then look at the list and see how well you did. Then do this again the next day but increase the images you are trying to remember up one digit, meaning 1-6. Repeat this exercise every day until you can fully recite all nine images before looking at the list.

After you have accomplished that, go shopping. Use the associations you acquired from your personal Major Method list to locate the items you want to buy.

Memory Enhancement Exercise 4: Study the Major Method List

Look up the Major Method on your own and study it very carefully. Take notes on it exactly as it appears. Then do the same exercise that you did with your own personal list but instead do it with the official Major Method list of number and letter associations. After you have memorized it, and associated images to every number/letter combination, go shopping like you did in exercise 3.

The Neuroscientist Technique

Chunking is when you take separate (chunks) of information and group them all together. Doing this will allow you to be able to take several disparate pieces of information and collect them together. You will be remembering only one collective whole instead of the sums of its parts. This is a valuable technique to know and is not very confusing.

This is a favorite technique of neuroscientist Daniel Bor. He came to realize how powerful a technique this was when he ran a test on an undergraduate volunteer who was only labeled to have an average IQ. He was read off random numbers and then asked to repeat them back in the order he heard them. When he succeeded, they would add an extra digit to the number sequence. When he failed, they would shorten the sequence by one. This test lasted two years and happened for an hour a day, four days out of the week.

It took an entire twenty months to see strong results, but by then the volunteer could recite back a number sequence that was 80 digits long. Daniel Bor had this to say about that.

"if 7 friends in turn rapidly told him their phone numbers, he could...key all 7 friends' numbers..."

The next time that you have a list and are required to recall items from it, use chunking to break everything up into smaller groups. An example would be having a list of words, like a vocabulary list, and first ordering the words that are related or similar to each other. Or if you have a shopping list then take a good look at it and take the first letter from each word and then combine them to make a chunked word.

An example would look like this; Donuts (D), Apples (A), Raisins (R), Eggs (E) are on your shopping list. Chunk together the first letters from every item and you will get the word "DARE". Instead of remembering every item all you will have to recall is the word "DARE".

Another method of chunking is relating the items on a list of things you have previous experience with. If you are buying things like eggs, and chocolate, then all you have to do is remember those cookies your grandmother used to bake for you when you were a child.

The area where chunking really starts to shine is when you are trying to remember a string of numbers, like a phone number. This can also work for a social security number or even computer passwords. You probably already do this and just don't notice. Let's pick a random string of numbers.

7598724418

Now, all we have to do to chunk it is add a few dashes and it will turn into this...

759-872-4418

As we mentioned earlier, the average person can hold about seven items in there STM. The above example has ten numbers listed which exceeds that amount. Yet by adding some dashes, we have broken up the long string into three separate chunks. Instead of having to remember all ten numbers separately, you only have to recall the three chunks.

Memory Enhancement Exercise 5: Remembering phone numbers

Start by asking people for their phone numbers. You don't have to ask strangers, ask people who you already know and have their phone numbers written down somewhere. Don't just ask them to tell you their phone numbers but have them write them down on a sheet of paper, but don't look at the paper. Just keep it for later. When they tell you the phone numbers, chunk them into groups of only three or four. Do this with two separate people a day. Later before you go to bed, recite those phone numbers and check the sheets they gave you to see how well you did. Also, be sure when they are first telling you their numbers, to recite them back out loud in chunks as that will help you to retain the information. Do this every day, with two people, until you can remember every new phone number by the end of the night for three days straight. Then you may move onto the next exercise.

Memory Enhancement Exercise 6: Chunking Random Numbers

This is exactly the same exercise as number 5, except it is only to be done on the spot in real life scenarios. There is no set routine to this exercise. Any time the chance to learn a string of numbers pops up, chunk them on the spot. Then later before going to bed, recite the string of numbers and see how well you did. Seeing as this is a real-world field exercise, there is no time limit for it. You can do this one for the rest of your life and keep on improving your memory.

The (beginner friendly) Ancient Greece Method

A Memory Palace is also known as "the method of loci". It stretches all the way back to the long-ago days of ancient Greece. Do not think that just because this technique is so old it has lost value though.

Boris Konrad is a memory champion, worldwide, and he not only uses the Memory Palace to win such championships but he along with Martin Dresler came together to perform a study on boosting memory, mainly using the Memory Palace as the cornerstone technique. Martin Dresler is a neuroscientist at a medical center university based in the Netherlands. Seeing as these are two authorities in the world of memory their study and findings shed much light on why the Memory Palace works so well.

Several different volunteers were divided into three groups. 23 of these people were memory competition regulars and 51 never competed in an official memory contest but did resemble them in age, intelligence, and health. Everyone had their brains scanned with FMRI (functional magnetic resonance imaging). At first, there was no clear distinction between anyone's brains, even when comparing the memory competitors against the non-memory competitor's.

Out of all these people, there was no noticeable increase in anyone's memory for those that did not do any memory training. This should come as no surprise. Another control group practiced basic concentration techniques. On average the people who practiced concentrating did see some slight improvements in their memory. Most of them could recall about 26 out of every 30 words they heard. After a period of practicing concentration techniques for 40 days, they could on average recall 11 more extra words.

The people in the third control group were practicing specific mnemonic techniques, such as the method of loci (Memory Palace). This group saw a huge boost to their memory power. A public platform called "Memocamp" was offered to them and was chosen by Dresler because it had been used by a variety of memory champions before. By the time the study was finished, the people in control group 3 had seemed to double the overall power of their memory within just 40 days.

That wasn't all though. When their brains were scanned using FMRI again, a surprising discovery was made. What was first noticed was that the overall blood flow to everyone's brain had increased. The second amazing discovery was that the brain activity of about 2,500 connections increased. Out of these 2,500 different areas of their brains, 25 of them stood out since they were all connected with being linked to the greater memory skills of the memory contest regulars and champions. All in all, the people of control group 3 were starting to develop brains similar to those who have the best memories on out planet.

"I think the most interesting part..." Dresler said after the study was concluded and he wanted to report the good news. "of our study is the comparison of these behavioral memory increases with what happens on the neurobiological level."

There you have it. Proof that if you put in the time and effort, then you can literally change the way your brain operates. Neuroplasticity gone right is capable of working wonders, along with the proper mindset and keeping a positive attitude while training. Yet Dresler had a bit more to say about the success of the study.

"By training this method...that all the memory champions use, your changeable brain connectivity patterns develop in the direction of the world's best memory champions."

But he also, as we have declared in this book, made it a clear point that no one will see results just from a one time practicing of these techniques.

"You do have to apply this for it to work…. Your memory doesn't just get better in general. So when you don't apply this strategy, probably your memory is only as good as it was before."

And memory champion Boris Konrad had this to say about the study.

"As it was my training paradigm we used…" He said. "and I have trained many groups with it before, I at least knew it does work-and work well."

Right from the horse's mouth you just heard the truth of how powerful maintaining the proper mindset is. This may sound trite, but if Boris Konrad and other random people who were involved with the study can do this, there is no reason why you should not be able to as well.

Building and Utilizing A Memory Palace

To build a Memory Palace you want to first select a real-world location that you are very familiar with, like your own home. Start right now. Close your eyes and imagine the home you currently live in (even if you are already there). You should notice that envisioning where you live already gives you many intrinsic details without having to push your imagination too hard. You should be able to see the colors of the walls, the arrangement of furniture, and everything else. Now, mentally, start walking around your home inside your mind. If you had trouble envisioning your home with your eyes closed then take more time and try it again. Being able to clearly see your home inside your mind's eye will be a valuable trait to develop before trying to utilize more of the Memory Palace. Take your time as you explore the Memory Palace of your home. Go from room to room. Turn the lights on and off. Take a look out the windows. Sit down on the couch. Go into the kitchen and cook some food. Then push it further by feeling your hands against the walls. Smell the food you are cooking. Feel the carpet underneath your feet. Take your time and get as detailed and comfortable as you can get.

The reason why you want to make everything as real and vivid as you can is that you will be returning to your Memory Palace quite often. As you go about your life you are going to store various memories inside your Memory Palace. This technique has even been replicated in movies and literature, like "Silence of the Lambs" or "Hannibal" and even (albeit indirectly) in Stephen King's Dark Tower novel series. So, it is not just for memory champions and neurological wizards.

The major premise behind establishing a Memory Palace is to associate specific areas of a familiar location (in this case your own home) with whatever general information you would like to remember why you live your life. As you traverse and explore your Memory Palace you are going to want to place mental constructs of various information inside of it. These should not be random things as much as they are specific concepts that you will want to remember and recall later.

An example of the Memory Palace in action would be if you knew you were going to meet with three different people tomorrow at different times. Let's say a lawyer at 9 AM, a client of yours at 2:30 PM, and your child's teacher at 4 PM. Before going off to see everyone place each one of them in your palace. You don't even need to know what they look like to accomplish this.

Place the lawyer at the front door of your (mental) home. Make him detailed. Dress him in a nice suit and add a briefcase in his hands. Have him knock on your door as if he was trying to get your attention. Go and greet him at the door, and when you open it and look at him, see that a tattoo saying "9 AM" is on his forehead.

Then go over to your couch. What's that? Someone is sitting on your couch and waiting for you. It's your client and he is wearing a shirt that clearly says "2:30 PM".

Then go over to your child's bedroom and take a peak inside. You should notice that there is a desk and a woman sitting behind it. She must be your child's teacher. Behind her is a backboard with "4 PM" written on it in chalk.

This is just a basic premise of how to construct your memory palace. You don't need to just use your palace for remembering appointments. You can also place people's names on their shirts, or anything else you want to recall about them.

If you would rather remember words instead then just get a little more creative. If you are supposed to later recall a message that one person asked you to give to another, find a place in your palace to store it. Go inside your bedroom, or wherever you want, and envision the message that you are supposed to relay scribbled all over your wall and making a mess of things. Tell yourself that, until you deliver the message, the graffiti is not going to be removed from your palace. After you have passed the message along, return to your mental bedroom and then discover that the walls have cleaned themselves up. That is the true power of linking real world memory to our imaginations- we can make a total mess of our palace and then sort it out later. There is no limit to what the human mind can do.

Memory Enhancement Exercise 7: Creating Your Memory World

You should have already started this just by learning what the Memory Palace is. You do not need to use your own home for your Memory Palace. You just need to make sure that whatever you select is something very familiar to you. It can be a stretch of a park or trail that you enjoy, an old job or home you used to have that you wouldn't mind mentally revisiting often, or anything else. Whatever you decide to construct your Memory Palace after, just make sure you are familiar with it on an intimate level. If you decide to really let your imagination run wild and create something entirely fictional that will be fine as well but make sure that whatever you chose is detailed down to every nook and cranny.

After deciding what you want your Memory Palace to be, visit it and explore for several minutes. Upon first visiting it, only place one simple memory inside of it. It is probably best to select something that is not important, but you still want to remember anyway.

An example would be; you are going to go to the store three days from now to buy a basketball. Granted you may not need one, but that is the point. We are using the basketball because it is something you don't need and may forget about. First, make a note on your calendar to revisit your palace in three days. Then go inside your palace.

Find a location in your palace to place the basketball. Let's say the driveway. You should see yourself literally begin to dribble the basketball while standing in the driveway, then walk away. As you walk away the ball should continue to bounce all on its own. Leave your palace and go about your day.

Three days later when you see marked on your calendar to revisit your palace you may have forgotten why, until you see the driveway and notice that a basketball is dribbling itself. Then you will remember to go to the store and buy the ball.

When doing this technique, the basketball is only an example. You should select a different object to use for this trick. Just make sure that it is not something so important when first practicing.

One Final Trick

How fun and impressive would it be if you were capable of memorizing an entire deck of cards? Yes, it may sound impossible but if you have made it this far then you should know that it can be done with the proper methods and state of mind.

This trick will contain many different aspects of everything you had learned thus far, so by practicing it you will be utilizing several different training methods at once.

First remove all the face cards (Kings, Queens, and Jacks from every suit) from the deck as those are all you will be working with at the start. There are a total of 12 face cards. Now associate a person you know with each card. They can be people you know in real life, athletes, celebrities, or even fictional characters. I like to use my own sister for the Queen of Clubs (please don't ask me why) and Bill Gates for the King of Diamonds (I assume he has a lot of diamonds). Now associate an action to the personality you gave to the card. For my sister, I associate her hitting things (again, please don't ask) and for Bill Gates, I associate him counting money. Now associate an object with the personalities and actions. For my sister, I associate a golf club, and for Bill Gates, I associate a diamond encrusted crown. Then recite this acronym in your head until it moves into your LTM...

PAO

It stands for...

P = Person
A = Action
O = Object

The reason for doing this is because you will be drawing three cards in a row after shuffling them. For whatever cards you draw follow the PAO formula when looking at them. The first card is the Person, the second is the Action, and the third is the Object. Continue to do this until you feel confident that no matter what face cards you draw, you will be able to remember the PAO formula for each one. You may not have realized it but following the PAO formula is actually a method of chunking information, though slightly different from the one used to recall a string of numbers. It is based on the same principle though.

We have my sister for the Queen of Clubs and Bill Gates for the King of Diamonds. For the Jack of Spades, I will associate it with my friend Jack (for obvious reasons). Now to push this further, we are going to want to place these images inside the Memory Palace.

I am going to place my sister, with her golf club, hitting the front door. I am going to place Bill Gates with his diamond encrusted crown sitting on the floor in my living room and counting his money. I am going to place my friend, Jack, with a spade, digging in the backyard.

You are going to want to do this with every one of the 12 face cards. This will take some time. If anyone ever told you that they could memorize an entire deck of cards in less then a minute, on the first try, without training first then they have lied to you. Don't bother trying to move onto the rest of the deck until you have found a place for every face card, following the PAO system, inside of your Memory Palace.

After you have gotten that far it is time to move onto the numbered cards. This may be harder to select associations for. Go through the entire deck and see if any images just naturally pop into your head for whatever reason. Does 4 of Hearts leap out at you and remind you of your cat? If you have a cat and you love the 4-legged little critter, then it just might. Or if you want to feel snazzy then just make yourself the Ace of Spades. There is nothing wrong with considering yourself as an Ace or a Spade. In fact, do that if you are feeling that you need a boost in confidence.

For the rest of the card you can use what is known as the "Dominic System" It looks like this...

1 = A

2 = B

3 = C

4 = D

5 = E

6 = S

7 = G

8 = H

9 = N

0= O

And for the suits...

Hearts = H

Spades =S

Diamonds = D

Clubs = C

For 2 of Clubs, you can associate the image of Brendan Fraser (he played a caveman in the movie "Encino Man") holding two archaic clubs in his hand and dancing like a fool (which he also did in the same movie) and place him wherever you want in your Memory Palace. Notice that for the 2 of Clubs we are still following the PAO system. The person is Brendan

Fraser , the action is dancing like a fool and the objects are the two-separate caveman like clubs.

These are all just examples of course. To truly get the hang of memorizing a deck of playing cards you will have to associate every card and image with things you are familiar with already.

Just getting the PAO for a single card may take a decent length of time and effort. That is why, while practicing this trick, you have to make it fun. This is one of the better parts about training your memory- you get to let your imagination run away as if you were a child once again. It can not be understated how important it is to make this exercise as fun as possible. Go ahead and let a series of utterly absurd images flood your mind. Let your imagination soar to heights that you have forgotten or never reached before. By the time you have memorized every card in the deck, you should have had such a good time doing it that you will almost be sad to have crossed the finish line.

Keep that mindset for every other tip and training exercise you have been given. Some of them will take great amounts of dedication and study, as they should since they are aimed to strengthen your concentration along with your memory. That shouldn't be the main focus though. It has been said that the goal is not more important then the journey. While increasing your memory, remember to enjoy yourself and let your (focused) imagination run wild as if you were young again. After all, that is what we are really training our brain to believe.

Memory Training Checklist

Due to the abundant amount of information in this book, having a handy go-to checklist to look at should help consolidate everything that you have to practice. Always try your best to understand that training of any sort is a long-term commitment. You will not see quick results if you do not put in the effort. Look at this checklist on a daily basis and keep logs of how well your memory is improving. It should also be stated that one thing we have not extolled enough about in the previous chapters has been getting the right amount of exercise. Regular exercise, especially of a cardio nature, will increase both blood flow and oxygen to your brain and help to make your memory even stronger. Along with exercise, you should highly consider introducing meditation into your life as well. Passively speaking, nothing will strengthen your concentration and memory like meditating.

- Make daily journal entries. Write down all your successes. Write down at least thee things a day that you found fulfillment or appreciation in.

- Practice calm meditation.

- Get regular amounts of exercise.

- Have your blood sugar levels checked?

- Get a hearing test.

- Floss twice daily.

- Find out your BMI and aim to keep it under 25.

- Envision yourself as a winner in every day life.

- Make sure you are getting enough vitamin B-12, but also make sure you are not just buying the first one you find.

- Eat the proper foods, especially leafy green vegetables, water, and plenty of fish.

- Learn how to use chopsticks and the etiquette involved with them.

- Have a routine set up before going to sleep. Also, have a set schedule to stay on throughout your day.

- Always try to think in terms of associations.
- Practice thinking in images and create clear visualizations in your head.
- Start playing with Rubik's cubes.
- Be mindful of your caffeine intake.
- Avoid sleeping medication that contains Diphenhydramine.
- Practice Memory Enhancement Exercise 1: Shopping with a Peg List
- Practice Memory Enhancement Exercise 2: Random Questions
- Practice Memory Enhancement Exercise 3: Creating Your Own List
- Practice Memory Enhancement Exercise 4: Study the Major Method List
- Practice Memory Enhancement Exercise 5: Chunk random Phone Numbers
- Practice Memory Enhancement Exercise 6: Chunking Random Numbers
- Practice Memory Enhancement Exercise 7: Creating Your Palace

- Memorize an entire deck of playing cards. It will take some time but be sure to keep at it until you can pull it off and have fun while doing it.
- NEVER GIVE UP!

Conclusion

Thank for making it through to the end of *How to Improve Your Memory After 40: Remember Everything and Stay Young*, let's hope it was informative and able to provide you with all of the tools you need to achieve your goals whatever they may be.

The next step is to put this book down and find something else to do. Exercise, meditate or even go play with a Rubik's cube. Separate yourself from all the material you just took in, then return to it later and see how much you remembered. Read it again, take notes, organize your priorities, and then get to work practicing all the techniques. After doing that for a week, read the book again and see if you remember even more then last time.

The techniques in this book must be practiced every day, or you will not see a powerful change. These lessons and techniques must be instilled into you on daily basis for neuroplasticity to take place and alter your current mind into the one you want. This will require effort and discipline, but when speaking of our memories and the mind, nothing is more important.

Also, please be sure to make appointments to get your hearing tested, figure out your blood sugar level, your BMI, floss daily, and make a list of attainable goals that you can reach today. Never forget you can change and its never too late to start!

Finally, if you found this book useful in any way, a review on Amazon is always appreciated!

Thanks,
John Gamberini